POCKET TRAINER FOR LEGS

21 Day Home Workout Guide
for Strong and Sexy Legs

Doug Bennett
TOP AMERICAN TRAINER

The Pocket Trainer for Legs is a day-by-day expert workout and diet guide you can do right at home to help you transform your entire lower body, boost energy, build endurance, increase strength and love your results in 21 days.

Each workout has 3 levels of intensity (beginner, intermediate and ultra-fit) that shapes, tones and sculpts your thighs, hips and bum. Plus, the diet plans included will double your chances of amazing success by kicking your slow metabolism into high gear to burn unwanted fat all day. In addition, each exercise has an expert description and pictorial on how to perform every exercise like a fitness pro.

Don't be frustrated any longer with those extra pounds you can't lose, workouts that don't work or the jiggly skin on your thighs and waist.

Let Doug Bennett, Top American Trainer and Developer of the former #4 ranked Fitgirl App on itunes, show you a solution to getting the amazing results you desire without paying thousands to train with an expert trainer.

The Pocket Trainer for Legs can be done at home, travel or at the gym. Now You don't have to wonder what exercises or workout to do to get tight inner thighs, lean legs, flat belly and a cute bum.

Is it challenging? Yes. This is not a 7 minute workout plan. Each workout is easy to follow and will help you smash calories while sculpting and toning muscle. You'll just need a few dumbbells, little motivation and this ultimate plan to start to see amazing changes in less than 7 days.

TABLE OF CONTENTS

Who this is not for: 1

The Medical Disclaimer: 2

Food Plans 3

3- Day Flush Diet **5**

    MEAL 1 (eat all) 5

    MEAL 2 5

    MEAL 3: 6

    MEAL 4 7

    MEAL 5 7

Get Results Diet **8**

    MEAL 1 9

    MEAL 2 9

    MEAL 3 10

    Protein (3-6 ounces choices below): 10

    *Greens (1-3 Cups choices below): 10

    *Veggies (1/2 -1 cup choices below): 11

    MEAL 4 11

    MEAL 5 12

**Handy List of All The Good Foods To Eat For Each Meal
that's Highlighted in Green for the "Get Results Diet."** **14**

    Good Carbs: 14

    Bad Carbs: 15

    Good Protein: 15

    Best Fruits (organic): 16

    Greens: 16

    Veggies: 16

    More Tips: 17

HOME Series Workouts **19**

WEEK 1 19

DAY 1 19
DAY 2 22
DAY 3 24
DAY 4 26
DAY 5 28
DAY 6 32
DAY 7 33

WEEK 2 34

DAY 1 34
DAY 2 36
DAY 3 38
DAY 4 41
DAY 5 43
DAY 6 47
DAY 7 48

WEEK 3 49

DAY 1 49
DAY 2 52
DAY 3 54
DAY 4 57
DAY 5 59
DAY 6 63
DAY 7 64

Exercise Pictorials and Descriptions: **65**

Summary: **86**

Check out my other books for more help: 86

WHO THIS IS NOT FOR:

This plan is not for someone who just wants to do a few squats, jumping jacks, lunges, etc. This is not like 99% of the plans that are copycat workouts that tell you "to do 10 of this and 10 of that" just to fill the paper with garbage.

"THIS IS A TAKE ACTION BOOK. NOT FOR READING!" - Doug Bennett

This is the most challenging workout that you can do with very little equipment. If you do love the gym, don't fret. Doug will be releasing a companion to this workout just for the gym. Yes, gym workouts are even more effective then home workout but Doug guarantees that **The Pocket Trainer for Legs** <u>at home</u> will give you better results than any program selling on Instagram for $69.00 - $99.00.

THE MEDICAL DISCLAIMER:

I'm not a doctor nor do I pretend to be. Always consult with your primary health care professional before starting any diet or fitness program. The material in this book, **The Pocket Trainer for Legs** written by Doug Bennett of The Body Studio Corp., is for informational purposes only. Use any of the information (diet, exercise and techniques) in this book at your own risk. Each individual needs vary from person to person. The information in this book is not a personal diet or exercise plan. The author, Doug Bennett, expressly disclaims responsibility for any injury or adverse effects that may be caused from the use or application of information in this book. Always stop exercising immediately and call for medical help if you feel dizzy, weak or faint.

Copyright:

So, are you ready to get going? Are you ready to dedicate yourself to eating only natural, low-fat foods? Are your ready to give your best to each workout? Well, if you answered yes to all these questions then expect results.

NOTE: this workout will take work. Nothing is worth it if you're not working for it.

Lets Go!

FOOD PLANS

Big changes and results will never happen without the right diet. Hence, I added 2 diets that I give to many of my clients to help them get the full benefit of using my training guides.

Most important diet tips are:

1. Eliminate refined sugars and preservatives.
2. Weigh out portions of foods if you're not getting better results.
3. If you're not hungry then don't eat snacks in between meals
4. Never eat till completely full.
5. Find meals that are easy to cook and stick to them until you drop any unwanted weight.
6. Don't eliminate all carbs but limit them to 1-2 per day (brown rice, wild rice, yams, potatoes, quinoa, oats). Make sure the portions are smaller.
7. One bad meal = 3 hard workouts
8. Fill up on organic greens and steamed veggies.
9. Refrain from alcohol or drink 1-2 glasses on the weekends only.
10. Drink water all day. Green tea and herbal teas are great.
11. Make sure your cabinets and fridge are stocked with the following:
    - Organic soups
    - Organic berries (blueberry and strawberries)
    - Green apples and Grapefruits
    - Organic carrots

- Raw seeds
- Organic oats or steel cut oats (instant)
- Frozen fruits and veggies (organic best)
- Spring water
- Sparkling water
- Herbal teas
- Free range broth (veggie and chicken)
- Hemp or natural whey protein
- Ezekiel bread and cereal (almond is best)
- Eggs
- Low-fat milk or unsweetened non-dairy beverage (hemp, almond, coconut)
- Free range meats (chicken on bone or breast, ground turkey or beef, lean cuts steak...limit to 2x week)
- Fish (light tuna in water or sunflower oil, white fish, salmon, shrimp)
- Raw nut butter
- Organic jam
- Greens (kale, spinach, mixed greens, alfalfa, arugula)
- Extra virgin olive oil, coconut oil and earth balance butter spread.
- Snacks: Organic Tortilla chips, Cedar's Hummus, Organic Dark Chocolate, raw nuts and dried fruit (2-3 ounces day)

Below are 2 diets: 3 Day Flush Diet (Day 1 -3) and Get Results Diet (Day 4 – 21).

These both will hopefully get you motivated to eat a clean whole foods lifestyle diet.

3- DAY FLUSH DIET

MEAL 1 (eat all)

- 16 ounces spring water with juice from fresh squeezed lemon
- 2 egg whites, hard boiled egg or 1/2 cup Ezekiel Almond Cereal with unsweetened, nondairy beverage (coconut or almond). Let soak for few minutes.
- ½ cup berries

Optional: add 6 ounces organic unsweetened Greek Yogurt if still hungry

MEAL 2

Green Drink (see recipes below)

Blend All (add 1 scoop natural vanilla whey or rice protein to each) :

1 Cup organic berries	½ cup cucumber
6-8 Spinach leaves	2 celery stalks
6-8 Kale leaves	6-8 Kale leaves
1/2 Cup Coconut Water or unsweetened coconut or almond milk	1/2 Cup pineapple
2 Tbsp. Wheat Germ	½ cup pear
1 small organic slightly ripe banana	¼ tsp cinnamon
1-2 Scoop protein	1 small organic slightly ripe banana
	1-2 Scoop Protein

1 cup organic carrot juice (premade)

½ cup frozen strawberries

6-8 Kale leaves

6 – 8 Spinach Leaves

1 small organic slightly ripe banana

1-2 Scoop Protein

¼ cup black berries

½ cup blueberries

6-8 Kale leaves

½ small avocado (ripe)

Tsp chia or hemp seeds

1 small organic slightly ripe banana

1-2 Scoop protein

MEAL 3:

Salad Bowl (Mix All):

- 2 cups Leafy Greens (kale, spinach, red leaf lettuce, dandelion, swiss chard, watercress, romaine, arugula
- 1 ounce raw nuts and/or seeds
- ½ cup Quinoa or Brown Rice (found in the frozen section of most health food stores, i.e. Trader Joes)
- 1 Tbsp. Avocado
- 1 Cup Chopped Organic Veggies (carrots, peppers, red onions, beets, celery, broccoli, radishes, cherry tomatoes, shredded cabbage, cucumbers, scallions)
- 2 tbsp. Dressing (just lemon juice, dressing below or Newman's Own Lite Dressings or Organic Vinegar and Oil)

DRESSING (MIX IN BLENDER, LOW):

- 2 cups Extra Virgin Olive Oil

- Juice from 1 whole organic lemon
- Pinch sea salt
- 1 teaspoon. Agave
- Small Handful chopped basil
- 1/8 cup red wine vinegar
- 1 tbsp. shredded parmesan or sheep cheese
- 1 tsp. dry mustard
- 2 Crushed Garlic Clove

MEAL 4

½ grapefruit or 1 cup watermelon or ½ cup organic berries (blackberries, strawberries, blueberries)

MEAL 5

1-2 Cups Broth Veggie Soup (low-fat veggie soup you love at Whole Foods, natural food section of your local grocery store or favorite recipe)

1-2 Cup Salad Greens (Kale, Spinach, Red Lettuce, Romaine) with 2 tbsp. dressing as above

½ cup Greek yogurt (unsweetened) or melon.

Still hungry late night ?

Eat ½ pink grapefruit or 1 cup watermelon

After 3 days of the "Fat Flush Diet", start with the " Get Results Diet" below.

GET RESULTS DIET

Mission: lose weight, tone and lean, increase energy and reach a lower fat percentage.

Eliminate all processed foods, chemicals, artificial sugars, hydrogenated fats and fatty meats. Eat only all natural. Increase protein. Consume little sugar and starch. Drink water at least 6x per day and take a daily probiotic vitamin and electrolyte supplement.

Daily Goal (Food Intake, servings): Greens (3-4), Lean Protein (3-4), Good Carbs (1), Good Fats (2-3), Fruits (2).

Fitness Goal:

60% cardio

- ➢ 30 minute (3-4 days): intermittent high intensity 90% max heart rate and 70% max heart rate
- ➢ 45 plus minutes (1 day): 60-75% max heart rate

40 % Resistance

- ➢ 3-4 days of weighted exercises: 4 - 6 circuits of your primary 2 body parts you want to change. Use heavier weights where needed (dumbbells) and add dumbbells to most exercises i.e. hip lifts, burpees….
- ➢ 1-2 days of body resistance: circuit push ups, pull ups, plyometrics (jumping, skipping), sprinting, mountain climbers, rope climbing, etc. 15-30 seconds each exercise x 5-12 circuits (no or 30 seconds rest between entire circuits)

MEAL 1

½ - 1 cup Fruit + 2-4 ounces Protein

- 1 Cup of fruit (blackberries, blueberries, strawberries) and hardboiled egg
- ½ pink grapefruit, 1 cup low-fat cottage cheese
- ½ cup fruit or ½ banana whipped into 1 cup Greek Yogurt (low-fat, unsweetened)
- 3 slices natural turkey bacon, green apple
- Protein Drink: ½ cup fruit, coconut or spring water, 2 scoops natural protein powder
- Sliced Apple, 1tbsp. raw almond butter, hard boiled egg
- 1 cup fresh fruit, 2 tbsp. wheat germ and ½ cup natural, Greek yogurt (unsweetened).

MEAL 2

½ cup Good Carb + tsp or 2 ounces Good Fat

- ½ cup rice (short grain brown rice, sprouted jasmine, wild rice) with tsp. oil (olive or coconut oil)
- Brown Rice Cake and tsp. raw nut butter (sunflower, almond, cashew, peanut)
- ½ cup sweet potato or red bliss potatoes (home fries) and tsp. Earth Balance Butter or Coconut Oil
- Slice Ezekiel Toast with 1 tsp natural hummus or avocado and slice tomato
- 1 low-fat mozzarella stick and ½ cup organic carrots
- Brown Rice cake, slice tomato and sprouts

- ½ cup celery or carrot sticks and 1 tsp. avocado or raw almond butter
- ½ cup Ezekiel Almond Cereal with 1 cup nondairy, unsweetened beverage (coconut or almond)

MEAL 3

<mark>Protein + Veggie + Salad</mark>

- ➢ 3-5 ounces protein
- ➢ 1-2 cups steamed, raw or sautéed veggies in broth
- ➢ 1 cup salad greens with fresh squeezed lemon juice

Protein (3-6 ounces choices below):

- o Light Tuna in water (wild caught, all natural with no preservatives)
- o Fish (wild salmon, shrimp, white fish, scallops)
- o Grass Fed, Organic: Chicken Breast, Ground Chicken & Turkey 85% lean, Turkey,
- o Grass Fed, Organic: Beef (top round, sirloin, flank), Ground Beef 85% lean, Ground Buffalo 85% lean
- o Tempeh, Tofu
- o Egg Whites

*Greens (1-3 Cups choices below):

- o Romaine Lettuce
- o Baby Kale
- o Baby Spinach and Red Spinach
- o Arugula

- o Red and Green Leaf Lettuce
- o Dandelion
- o Swiss Chard

*Veggies (1/2 -1 cup choices below):

- o Broccoli
- o Red Onions
- o Beets (roasted)
- o Peppers
- o Asparagus
- o Green Beans
- o Carrots
- o Tomatoes (fruit)
- o Artichoke Hearts
- o Asparagus
- o Edamame
- o Brussel Sprouts
- o Cabbage
- o Cauliflower
- o Leeks
- o Celery
- o Turnips
- o Zucchini
- o Cucumber

MEAL 4

½ cup – 1 cup Fruit + 2-4 ounces Protein

Protein Smoothie

1 cup favorite fruit, ½ cup unsweetened Greek Yogurt (optional), 2 scoops natural protein powder and unsweetened organic low-fat milk or nondairy beverage (coconut and/or almond). Blend to taste.

MEAL 5

Protein + Greens + Veggie

- ➢ 4-6 ounces Protein
- ➢ 1 – 2 Cups Greens with Lemon Juice
- ➢ ½-1 Cup Veggies

Or

See below for suggestions.

Clean Dinner Suggestions (fewer the ingredients the better):

- Ground Protein (organic beef, buffalo, chicken or turkey) mixed with sautéed veggies.
- 3-6 ounces White Fish baked in tinfoil with lemon juice, white wine and black pepper. Served with greens and stir fried veggies.
- 3-5 ounces Grilled Free Range Chicken sliced and placed on greens with veggies and Newman's Own Lite Caesar Dressing.
- Ground Protein (organic beef, buffalo, chicken or turkey) mixed with fresh pico de gallo over lettuce and pinch or natural Mexican shredded cheese (Cabot).
- 4-6 ounces Grilled Wild Salmon topped with chopped cucumber, avocado, tomato and lemon juice. Serve with wedge of Pink Grapefruit and salad.

- Scrambled Egg Whites with light cheese and turkey bacon. Two slices tomato and salad with veggies.
- 4-6 ounces Grilled Chicken topped with Bruschetta. Served with steamed asparagus and spinach.
- Organic Bone Broth Chicken Soup with veggies. Served with salad.
- Organic Veggie Broth Soup. Served with quinoa, raw nuts and lentils.
- Tofu sautéed in coconut oil with sliced carrots, chopped onion, garlic clove, cubed sweet potato and seasoning (curry, sea salt and cumin). Served with quinoa, raw nuts and lentils.
- Veggie Chili (lentils, white beans) in a tomato broth with sautéed carrots, onions and peppers. Add tofu or organic ground protein.

Late Night Snack (select one only if needed)

- ½ cup natural Greek Yogurt
- ½ cup berries
- 8 ounce protein drink

HANDY LIST OF ALL THE GOOD FOODS TO EAT FOR EACH MEAL THAT'S HIGHLIGHTED IN GREEN FOR THE "GET RESULTS DIET."

Good Carbs:

- Short Grain Brown Rice or Wild Rice
- Quinoa
- Yams
- Root Veggies
- Organic Whole or Steel Cut Oats
- Organic Oat Bran
- Lentils or Legumes
- Barley
- Brown Rice Pasta (Tinkyada Brand Only)
- Wheat Berry
- Sprouted Grains
- Sour Dough (sparingly: slice 1x week)
- Ezekiel Bread
- Buckwheat noodles
- Brown Rice Cakes (Lunberg brand)

Bad Carbs:

- Flour (all flour in general. Yet, if you need to bake use almond flour)
- Refined Sugars (molasses, brown sugar, table sugar, etc.. or any Baked Goods)
- Honey (unless raw and sparingly)
- Candy (natural or unnatural)
- Gum (sugar free included)
- Protein Bars (exceptions to eat sparingly)
- White Pasta or Rice (1/2 cup of each sparingly ok)
- Pizza Dough
- Cereals other then Ezekiel or Natures Path occasionally (brand flakes)

Cereals: make sure 4-6 grams fiber, less than 4 grams of simple sugar and low-fat. Plus, never more then 4-6 ingredients. Oatmeal with added oat bran and seeds (chia, flax or hemp) is best choice.

Good Protein:

- Fish
- Free Range lean Meats (chicken, buffalo, beef, turkey)
- Lentils and Brown Rice
- Seeds (hemp, chia, flax, sunflower) and Raw Nuts (almond, cashew, pistachio etc.)
- Protein Powders (hemp, pea, rice, natural whey)

Best Fruits (organic):

- Strawberries
- Blueberries
- Watermelon
- Green Apples
- Grapefruit
- Tomatoes

Greens:

- Kale
- Spinach
- Dandelion
- Arugula
- Mustard Greens
- Red lettuce

Veggies:

- Peppers
- Organic Assorted Carrots
- Asparagus
- Broccoli
- Shitake Mushrooms
- Red Onion
- Garlic
- Squash
- Spinach
- Zucchini

- Cucumber
- Cauliflower
- Celery
- Cabbage

More Tips:

✓ **Always eat** all natural and whole foods for a long term plan.

✓ **Eat smaller** portions.

✓ **Make sure lean protein in 3-4 meals**, 3-5 ounces if you are lifting weights.

✓ **Eat at home** or know where you'll eat (healthy options).

✓ **Stay away from** prepared frozen diet meals at your local supermarket (national brands).

✓ **Calories matter** so make sure you try to burn off more than you take in if you're trying to lose weight. Increase activity.

✓ **Drink spring water and green tea** (loose leaf) as much as possible.

✓ **It's Ok to eat a meal high in fat once in a while.** Eat less and make sure all natural.

✓ **Use many** herbs and spices for taste.

✓ **If you cheat with a high carb meal. Lift the next day and cut all carbs for that day.**

✓ **The Cleaner your foods** the leaner you'll get.

✓ **Find 3-4 of your favorite recipes** for protein, veggies and salads. Double the recipe and store for later in the week.

✓ **Warm tea and natural seltzer water** can help void cravings.

✓ **Food Prep and making sure your fridge and cabinets are stocked** with healthy foods are both key to eating a clean diet.

✓ **Track your fitness and calories** with a fitness tracker (i.e. Fitbit)

HOME SERIES WORKOUTS

WEEK 1

Day 1

Exercises	Beginner	Intermediate	Fit Girl
Jump Rope or Jumping Jacks	1 minute	3 minutes	3 minutes with intermediate high knee running, every 30 seconds for 30 seconds
Squats : Legs	Air squats 25 reps	Air squats 25 reps	Air squats 25 reps
Bicycle : Abs	30 seconds	1 minute	1 minute
Squats	Air squats 25 reps	Dumbbell or Bar squats 15 reps w single dumbbell : 15-25 lbs. or 25lb. bar with weight	Dumbbell squats 15 reps w single dumbbell : 15-25 lbs. or 25lb. bar with weight
Bicycle : Abs	30 seconds	1 minute	1 minute
Squats	Air squats 25 reps	Dumbbell or Bar squats 15 reps w single dumbbell : 15-25 lbs. or 25lb. bar with weight	Dumbbell squats 15 reps w single dumbbell : 15-35 lbs. or 25lb. bar with weight
Bicycle : Abs	30 seconds	1 minute	1 minute
Bicycle with straight leg : Abs	30 seconds	1 minute	1 minute

Squats		Dumbbell or Bar squats 15 reps w single dumbbell : 15-25 lbs. or 25lb. bar with weight	Dumbbell squats 15 reps w single dumbbell : 15-45 lbs. or 25lb. bar with weight
Bicycle with straight leg : Abs	30 seconds	1 minute	1 minute
Squats followed by plie squat pulses		Dumbbell squats 15 reps w single dumbbell : 15-25 lbs. or 25lb. bar with weight immediately follow with 30 plie pulses	Dumbbell squats 15 reps w/ single dumbbell: 15-40 lbs. or 25lb. bar with weight immediately follow with 50 plie pulses
Jumping squats	10 reps	25 reps	25 reps
Star Jumps	10 reps	25 reps	25 reps
Plie' Pulse Squats or Plie Pulse Squats with a Dumbbell (15-25lbs.)	20 reps	50 reps	50 reps till failure
Skating	30 seconds	1 minute	1 minute
Walking Lunges 20 feet	1 minute: Holding no weight	1 minute: Holding no weight	1 minute: Holding no weight
Bicycle with straight leg : Abs	30 seconds	1 minute	1 minute
Walking Lunges 20 feet	Rest 1-2 minutes and proceed to plank	1 minute: Holding a dumbbell in each hand, 10-15lbs.	1 minute: Holding a dumbbell in each hand, 10-15lbs.

Exercise Pictorials and Descriptions

Skating	Rest	1 minute	1 minute
Plank	1 minute	1 minute with walking feet	1 minute with walking feet
Jumping Squats	Proceed to walk or run.	25 reps	25 reps holding weight (single dumbbell or medicine ball at chest level
Star Jumps	------	50 reps	50 reps
Push Ups	------	25-50 reps, start no knees	25-50 reps, start no knees
High Plank		1 minute with walking feet	1 minute with walking feet
Power Walk or Run	15 minutes	15 – 30 minutes	15 – 30 minutes, pick up the pace every other minute for 15 seconds

DAY 2

Exercises	Beginner	Intermediate	Fit Girl
Jump Rope or Jumping Jacks	1 minutes	3 minutes	3 minutes with intermediate high knee running, every 30 seconds for 30 seconds
Bridges	25 reps	50 with weight	50 with weight
One Leg Bridge	10 both side	25 both side w/ weight	25 both side w/ weight
Jump Rope or Jumping Jacks	1 minute	3 minutes	3 minutes with intermediate high knee running, every 30 seconds for 30 seconds
Bridges	25 reps	50 with weight	50 with weight
One Leg Bridge	10 both side	25 both side w/ weight	25 both side w/ weight
Push Ups	10 reps	25 reps	25 reps
Mountain Climbers, hit the ground with both balls of feet at same time!	30 seconds	1 minute	1 minute
Bridges	25 reps	50 with weight	50 with weight
One Leg Bridge	10 both side	25 both side w/ weight	25 both side w/ weight
Mountain Climbers, hit the ground with both balls of feet at same time!	30 seconds	1 minute	1 minute

Jump Rope or Jumping Jacks	1 minutes	3 minutes	3 minutes with intermediate high knee running, every 30 seconds for 30 seconds
Bridges	25	50 with weight	50 with weight
One Leg Bridge	10 both side	25 both side w/ weight	25 both side w/ weight
Swimming	30 seconds	1 minute	1 minute
Skating	1 minute	2 minutes	2 minutes
Back Leg Curl with Fitness Ball	15 reps	25 reps	25 reps
Stiff Leg Deadlifts with dumbbells	10 reps w/ 5-10 lbs.	10 reps w/15 lbs.	10 reps w/15 lbs.
Skating	Rest	1 minute	1 minute
Back Leg Curl with Fitness Ball	15 reps	25 reps	25 reps
Stiff Leg Deadlifts with dumbbells	skip	10 reps w/15 lbs.	10 reps w/15 lbs.
Swimming	30 seconds	1 minute	1 minute
Back Leg Curl with Fitness Ball	15 reps	25 reps	25 reps
Stiff Leg Deadlifts with dumbbells	Skip	10 reps w/15 lbs.	10 reps w/15-20 lbs.
Plank with walking	30 seconds	1 minute	1 minute
Push Ups w/ or w/out knees	30 seconds	1 minute or till failure	1 minute or till failure
Power Walk or Run	15 minutes	15 – 30 minutes	15 – 30 minutes, pick up the pace every other minute for 15 seconds

DAY 3

Exercises	Beginner	Intermediate	Fit Girl
Jump Rope or Jumping Jacks	1 minute	3 minutes	3 minutes with intermediate high knee running, every 30 seconds for 30 seconds
High Knee Running	30 Seconds	1 minute	2 minutes
Alternate Front Kicks, ball of foot	1 minute	2 minutes	2 minutes
Burpees	10 reps	25 reps	25 reps
Star Jumps	20 reps	50 reps	50 reps
Jump Rope or Jumping Jacks	1 minute	3 minutes	3 minutes with intermediate high knee running, every 30 seconds for 30 seconds
Leg Lifts : Abs	10 reps	50 reps	50 reps
High Knee Running	1 minute	2 minutes	2 minutes, increase pace for 15 seconds every 30 seconds
Skating	30 seconds	2 minutes	2 minutes
Switch kicks	1 minute	2 minutes	2 minutes
Burpee w/ Star	10 reps	25 reps	25 reps
Push Ups	10 reps	25-50 reps	25-50 reps
Abs : Leg Lifts Leg Lift Flutters	10 reps 15 seconds	50 reps 30 seconds	50 reps 30 seconds – 1 minute
Star Jumps	10 reps	25 reps	50 reps
Skating	30 seconds	1 minute	1 – 2 minutes
Stand Ups	5 each leg	25 each leg	25 each leg

			Optional: hold a medicine ball or dumbbell to chest under chin
Lunge pulses	10 reps each leg	25 each leg holding dumbbells in each hand (10-20lbs.)	25 each leg holding dumbbells in each hand (10-20lbs.)
Jump Rope or Jumping Jacks	1 minute	2 minutes	2 minutes with intermediate high knee running, every 30 seconds for 30 seconds
Lunge pulses	10 reps each leg	25 each leg holding dumbbells in each hand (10-20lbs.)	25 each leg holding dumbbells in each hand (10-20lbs.)
Leg Lifts : Abs	20 reps	50 reps	50 reps
Plank	1 minute	1 minute with walking feet	1 minute with walking feet
Standing Bicep Curls	20 reps, 5-10lbs.	25 reps, 10-15 lbs.	25 reps, 10-15lbs.
High Knee Running	------	1 minute	1 minute, intensity last 30 seconds
Push Ups	------	25-50 reps, start no knees	25-50 reps, start no knees
Stationary Lunge with dumbbell bicep curls	------	30 reps, switch legs every 15 reps	30 reps, switch legs every 15 reps
Power Walk or Run	15 minutes	15 – 30 minutes	15 – 30 minutes, pick up the pace every other minute for 15 seconds

DAY 4

Exercises	Beginner	Intermediate	Fit Girl
Jump Rope or Jumping Jacks	1 minute	3 minutes	3 minutes with intermediate high knee running, every 30 seconds for 30 seconds
Burpees	10 reps	20 reps	20 reps
Push Ups	5 reps	10 reps	10 reps
~~Burpees~~	10 reps	30 reps	30 reps
Push Up Pulses	10 reps	30 reps	50 reps
Burpees	5 reps	40 reps	50 reps
Bicycle : Abs	30 sec - 1 minute	1 minute	2 minutes
High Knee Running	1 minute	2 minutes	2 minutes, increase pace for 15 seconds every 30 seconds
1. Push Backs, dumbbells (pyramid) 10 reps light >>10 reps heavier>>5 reps heavier	5lbs>>8lbs>>10lbs (5rep>10rep5reps)	10lbs>>12lbs>>15-20lbs (5rep>10rep>5reps)	10lbs>>12lbs>>15-20lbs (5rep>10rep>5reps)
2. Push Ups	5 reps	10 reps	10 reps
3. Tricep Bench	10 reps	20 reps	20-30 reps
4. Star Jumps	10 reps	25 reps	25 reps

Repeat 1 to 4 above as directed before proceeding to bicycle	2 x	3 x	4-5 x
Bicycle : Abs	30 seconds	1 minute	1 minute
Knee Tucks : Abs	10 reps	25 reps	50 reps
Jump Rope or Jumping Jacks	1 minute	3 minutes	3 minutes with intermediate high knee running, every 30 seconds for 30 seconds
Power Walk or Run	30 minutes, Treadmill walk incline of 6-10 for 2 minutes every 3 minutes	30-45 minutes Treadmill jog incline 3-5 for 30 seconds every 5 minutes	30-45 minutes Treadmill jog incline 3-5 for 30 seconds every 5 minutes

DAY 5

Exercises	Beginner	Intermediate	Fit Girl
Jump Rope or Jumping Jacks	1 minute	3 minutes	3 minutes with intermediate high knee running, every 30 seconds for 30 seconds
Squats : Legs	Air squats 25 reps	Air squats 25 reps	Air squats 25 reps
Bicep Curls	Band 30 seconds or 5-10 lb. dumbbells 15 reps	Band 1 minute or 10-12 lb. dumbbells 15 reps	Band 1 minute or 10-12 lb. dumbbells 15 reps
Squats : Legs Follow with stand ups	Air squats 25 reps immediately follow with 5 stand ups each leg	Dumbbell or Bar squats 15 reps w single dumbbell : 15-25 lbs. or 25lb. bar with weight immediately follow with 20 stand ups each leg	Dumbbell squats 15 reps w single dumbbell : 15-25 lbs. or 25lb. bar with weight immediately follow with 20 stand ups each leg
Bicep Curls	Band 30 seconds or 5-10 lb. dumbbells 15 reps	Band 1 minute or 10-12 lb. dumbbells 15 reps. Best if you **pyramid (drop set) weight, change weight every 5 reps from heaviest to lighter but should challenge you.**	Band 1 minute or 10-12 lb. dumbbells 15 reps. Best if you **pyramid (drop set) weight, change weight every 5 reps from heaviest to lighter but should challenge you.**

		Example, 5-8 reps 15lbs drop and do 6-8 more reps with 12lbs. Challenge yourself safely with good form with heavier.	Example, 5-8 reps 15lbs drop and do 6-8 more reps with 12lbs. Challenge yourself safely with good form with heavier.
Squats : Legs	Air squats 25 reps	Dumbbell or Bar squats 25 reps w single dumbbell : 15-25 lbs. or 25lb. bar with weight. **Pyramid (drop set) weight heavy to light every 5-10 reps**	Dumbbell or Bar squats 25 reps w single dumbbell : 15-25 lbs. or 25lb. bar with weight. **Pyramid (drop set) weight heavy to light every 5-10 reps**
Walking Lunges 20 feet	Rest 1-2 minutes and proceed to plank	2 minute: Holding a dumbbell in each hand, 10-15lbs. Start out with Heaviest weight you can and every 20 feet drop to little lighter	2 minute: Holding a dumbbell in each hand, 10-15lbs. Start out with Heaviest weight you can and every 20 feet drop to little lighter
Bicep Curls	Band 30 seconds or 5-10 lb. dumbbells 15 reps	Band 1 minute or 10-12 lb. dumbbells 15 reps	Band 1 minute or 10-12 lb. dumbbells 15 reps
Squats : Legs	Air squats 25 reps	Dumbbell or Bar squats 25 reps w single dumbbell : 15-25 lbs. or 25lb. bar with weight.	Dumbbell or Bar squats 25 reps w single dumbbell : 15-25 lbs. or 25lb. bar with weight.

		Pyramid (drop set) weight heavy to light every 5-10 reps	Pyramid (drop set) weight heavy to light every 5-10 reps
Sissy Squats	25 reps	50 reps	100 reps
Bicep Curls	Band 30 seconds or 5-10 lb. dumbbells 15 reps	Band 1 minute or 10-12 lb. dumbbells 15 reps	Band 1 minute or 10-12 lb. dumbbells 15 reps
High Knee Step Ups	10 reps each leg	10 reps each leg holding a dumbbell in each hand 10-20 lb.	10 reps each leg holding a dumbbell in each hand 10-20 lb.
Squat and press (shoulder)	10 reps with 3-5 lbs.	20 reps with 3-8 lbs.	15 reps with 5-15 lbs.
High Knee Step Ups	10 reps each leg	10 reps each leg holding a dumbbell in each hand 10-20 lb.	10 reps each leg holding a dumbbell in each hand 10-20 lb.
Sissy Squats	25 reps	50 reps	100 Reps
High Knee Step Ups	Proceed to bridges	15 reps each leg holding a dumbbell in each hand 10-20 lb.	15 reps each leg holding a dumbbell in each hand 10-20 lb.
Bridges	25 reps	100 reps	100 reps
Single Leg Bridges	10 each leg	25 each leg	25 each leg
Jumping squats	10 reps	15-20 reps holding a dumbbell or medicine ball (15-25lb.) landing and going into full squat and jumping	15-25 reps holding a dumbbell or medicine ball (15-25lb.) landing and going into full squat and jumping

Exercise Pictorials and Descriptions

		up high with straight legs	up high with straight legs
Bridges	25 reps	100 reps	100 reps
Mile Run	Walk ½ mile and trot ½ mile	Jog ½ mile and 70% sprint ½ mile	Jog ½ mile and 70 % sprint ½ mile
Walk or run	Walk 15-30 minutes. Hill path. If you have a Treadmill walk incline 6-10.	Sprints (rest 30 sec between sets) 3 x 25 yards, 80% max 2 x 50 yards, same 1 x 100 yards, same	Sprints (rest 30 sec between sets) 3 x 25 yards, 80% max 2 x 50 yards, same 1 x 100 yards, same 2 x 50 yards, same

DAY 6

Exercises	Beginner	Intermediate	Fit Girl
Cardio	Power Walk, Bike and/or Run 2-4 miles	Run 4-5 miles Hills included	Run 4-6 miles Hills included
Abs: Knee Tucks	10 reps	25 reps	50 reps
Abs: Plank with walking	Plank with walking, 10 each side	Plank with walking, 20 each side	Plank with walking, 30 each side
Abs: High Plank to Low Plank	5 each side	15 each side	25 each side
Abs: Leg Lifts	10 reps	25 reps	50 reps
Abs: Side Plank	30 sec right and left side	1 minute right and left side	1 minute right and left side
Abs: Knee Tucks	10 reps	25 reps	50 reps
Cardio	Jump Rope or Jumping Jacks 2 minutes	Jump Rope or Jumping Jacks 3 minutes	Jump Rope or Jumping Jacks 3 minutes, every 30 seconds high knee running for 30 seconds

DAY 7

Rest and Stretch 20 minutes. Yoga is best.

WEEK 2

Day 1

Exercises	Beginner	Intermediate	Fit Girl
Jump Rope or Jumping Jacks	1 minute	3 minutes	3 minutes with intermediate high knee running, every 30 seconds for 30 seconds
Squats : Legs	Air squats 25 reps	Air squats 25 reps	Air squats 25 reps
Bicycle : Abs	30 seconds	1 minute	1 minute
Squats	Air squats 40 reps	Dumbbell or Bar squats 15 reps w single dumbbell : 15-25 lbs. or 25lb. bar with weight	Dumbbell squats 15 reps w single dumbbell : 15-25 lbs. or 25lb. bar with weight
Bicycle : Abs	30 seconds	1 minute	1 minute
Squats	Air squats 40 reps	Dumbbell or Bar squats 15 reps w single dumbbell : 15-25 lbs. or 25lb. bar with weight	Dumbbell squats 15 reps w single dumbbell : 15-35 lbs. or 25lb. bar with weight
Bicycle : Abs	1 minute	1 minute	1 minute
Bicycle with straight leg : Abs	30 seconds	1 minute	2 minutes
Squats	skip	Dumbbell or Bar squats 15 reps w single dumbbell : 15-25 lbs. or 25lb. bar with weight	Dumbbell squats 15 reps w single dumbbell : 15-45 lbs. or 25lb. bar with weight
Cross Overs	10 each side	25 each side	25 each side

Squats	skip	Dumbbell squats 15 reps w single dumbbell : 15-25 lbs. or 25lb. bar with weight	Dumbbell squats 15 reps w/ single dumbbell: 15-40 lbs. or 25lb. bar with weight
Jumping squats	15 reps	25 reps	25 reps
Star Jumps	10 reps	40 reps	50 reps
Squats		Dumbbell or Bar squats 10 reps w single dumbbell : 15-25 lbs. or 25lb. bar with weight	Dumbbell squats 15 reps w/ single dumbbell: 20-40 lbs. or 25lb. bar with weight
Skating	1 minute	2 minutes	2 minutes
Walking Lunges 20 feet	1 minute: Holding no weight	1 minute: Holding 10-15 lb. dumbbells	2 minutes: Holding 10-15 lb. dumbbells
Lunge Pulses	10 each leg	25 each leg	50 each leg
Cross Overs	10 each side	25 each side	25 each side
Sissy Squats	25 reps	50 reps	100 reps
Skating	Rest	1 minute	1 minute
Knee tucks	10-20 reps	25-50 reps	40-50 reps
Reverse Lunge with kicks	Skip	Each side 1 minute	Each side 1 minute
Sissy Squats	25 reps	50 reps	100 reps
Lunge Pulses	10 each leg	25 each leg	50 each leg
Push Ups	------	25-50 reps, start no knees	25-50 reps, start no knees
High Plank Arm Pulses		50 reps	50-100 reps
Power Walk or Run	15 minutes	15 – 30 minutes	15 – 30 minutes, pick up the pace every other minute for 15 seconds

DAY 2

Exercises	Beginner	Intermediate	Fit Girl
Jump Rope or Jumping Jacks	2 minutes	3 minutes	3 minutes with intermediate high knee running, every 30 seconds for 30 seconds
Bridges	50 reps	50 with weight	50 with weight
One Leg Bridge	20 both side	50 both side no weight	50 both side w/ weight
Mountain Climbers, hit the ground with both balls of feet at same time!	1 minute	2 minutes	2 minutes
Bridges	25 reps	50 with weight	50 with weight
One Leg Bridge	10 both side	50 both side w/ weight	50 both side w/ weight
Push Ups	10-20 reps	25-40 reps	25-50 reps
Heavy Plie Squats	15 reps, hold 15lbs	20 reps, hold 20-40 lbs.	25 reps, hold 20-50 lbs.
Bridges	25 reps	50 with weight	50 with weight
Stiff Leg Dead Lifts	10 with light weight 10-12lbs	15 with 10-20 lbs.	15 with 10-20 lbs.
Heavy Plie Squats, single dumbbell	15 reps w/ 15 lbs.	20 reps w/20-30 lbs.	25 reps w/20-40 lbs.
Skating	1 minute	2 minutes	2 minutes
Bridges	25	50 with weight	50 with weight
One Leg Bridge	10 both side	25 both side w/ weight	25 both side w/ weight

Back Leg Curl with Fitness Ball	10 reps	25 reps	25 reps
Swimming	1 minute	2 minutes	2 minutes
Heavy Plie Squats, single dumbbell followed by plie pulses (hands on thighs)	15 reps w/ 15 lbs. then follow with plie pulses 20 reps	20 reps w/20-30 lbs. then follow with plie pulses 50 reps	25 reps w/20-40 lbs. then follow with plie pulses 50 reps till failure
Stiff Leg Deadlifts with dumbbells	skip	10 reps w/15 lbs.	10 reps w/15 lbs.
Skating	skip	1 minute	1 minute
Back Leg Curl with Fitness Ball	10 reps	25 reps	25 reps
Stiff Leg Deadlifts with dumbbells	10 reps w/ 5-10 lbs.	10 reps w/15 lbs.	10 reps w/15 lbs.
Swimming	30 seconds	1 minute	2 minutes
Jumping Squat holding a medicine ball or dumbbell	10 reps, 5-10 lb.	15 reps,15-20 lb.	25 reps, 15-30 lb.
Stiff Leg Deadlifts with dumbbells	Skip	10 reps w/15 lbs.	10 reps w/15-20 lbs.
Skating	Skip	1 minute	1 minute
Push Ups w/ or w/out knees	30 seconds	1 minute or till failure	1 minute or till failure
Power Walk or Run	20 minutes	20- 30 minutes	20- 30 minutes, pick up the pace every other minute for 15 seconds

DAY 3

Exercises	Beginner	Intermediate	Fit Girl
Jump Rope or Jumping Jacks	2 minute	3 minutes	3 minutes with intermediate high knee running, every 30 seconds for 30 seconds
High Knee Running	2 minute	3 minutes	3 minutes, every 30 seconds perform 20 punches from your face in a boxing position
Switch kicks, ball of foot	1 minute	2 minutes	2 minutes
Reverse Lunge with kicks	15 reps each side	25 reps each side	30 reps each side
Star Jumps	25 reps	50 reps	50 reps
Mountain Climbers	1 minute	2 minutes	2 minutes, every 15 seconds perform 2 push ups
Leg Flutters 3 inches off the ground : Abs	Flutter 15 sec Criss cross 15 sec Repeat both 2x	Flutter 30 sec Criss Cross 30 sec Repeat both 2x	Flutter 30 sec Criss Cross 30 sec Repeat both 2x
45 Degree Crunches	10 reps	10 reps, draw in knees and repeat 3x	10 reps, draw in knees and

			repeat 4x
Skating	30 seconds	2 minutes	2 minutes
Alternate Front Kicks, ball of foot	1 minute	2 minutes	2 minutes
Burpees w/ star	10 reps	25 reps	25 reps
Push Ups	10 reps	25-50 reps	25-50 reps
Leg Lifts : Abs	20 reps	50 reps	50 reps
Star Jumps	10 reps	25 reps	50 reps
Jump Rope or Jumping Jacks	1 minute	2 minutes	2 minutes with intermediate high knee running, every 30 seconds for 30 seconds
Skating	30 seconds	1 minute	1 minute holding a dumbbell or medicine ball at chest
Stationary Lunge with bicep curls	20 reps, switch legs every 10 reps	30 reps, switch legs every 15 reps	30 reps, switch legs every 15 reps
Hammer curls	15 reps, 5-12 lbs	20 reps, 10-15 lbs.	20 reps, pyramid weight starting with heavy 15-20 lbs doing as many as possible and switch to lighter ie. 12lbs.
Stationary Lunge with	20 reps, switch legs every 10	30 reps, switch legs every 15 reps	30 reps, switch legs every 15

dumbbell bicep curls	reps		reps
Leg Lifts : Abs	20 reps	50 reps	50 reps
Plank	1 minute	1 minute with walking feet	1 minute with walking feet
Standing Bicep curls, curl together	15 reps, 8-12 lbs.	20 reps, pyramid weight starting with heavy 15-20 lbs doing as many as possible and switch to lighter ie. 12lbs.	20 reps, pyramid weight starting with heavy 15-20 lbs doing as many as possible and switch to lighter ie. 12lbs.
High Knee Running	------	1 minute	1 minute, intensity last 30 seconds
Push Ups	------	25-50 reps, start no knees	25-50 reps, start no knees
Stationary Lunge	------	20 reps each leg	25 reps each leg
Power Walk or Run	15 minutes	15 – 30 minutes	15 – 30 minutes, pick up the pace every other minute for 15 seconds

DAY 4

Exercises	Beginner	Intermediate	Fit Girl
Jump Rope or Jumping Jacks	1 minute	3 minutes	3 minutes with intermediate high knee running, every 30 seconds for 30 seconds
Burpees	10 reps	20 reps	20 reps
Push Ups	10 reps	20 reps	30 reps
Burpees w 10 high knee runs	10 reps	30 reps	30 reps
Push Up Pulses	20 reps	50 reps	50 - 100 reps
Burpees	5 reps	40 reps	50 reps
Bicycle : Abs	30 sec - 1 minute	1 minute	2 minutes
Sit ups with a twist	25 reps	25 – 50 reps	25 -50 reps
High Knee Runnlng	1 minute	2 minutes	2 minutes, increase pace for 15 seconds every 30 seconds
5. Push Backs, dumbbells (pyramid) 20 reps light >>15 reps heavier>>10 reps heavier	5lbs>>8lbs>>10lbs	10lbs>>12lbs>>15-20lbs	10lbs>>12lbs>>15-20lbs
6. Push Ups	10 reps	10 reps	10 reps
7. Tricep Bench	10 reps	20 reps	20-30 reps
8. Star Jumps	10 reps	25 reps	25 reps

Exercise Pictorials and Descriptions

Repeat 1 to 4 above as directed before proceeding to bicycle	2 x	3 x	4-5 x
Bicycle : Abs	30 seconds	1 minute	1 minute
Knee Tucks : Abs	10 reps	25 reps	50 reps
Jump Rope or Jumping Jacks	1 minute	3 minutes	3 minutes with intermediate high knee running, every 30 seconds for 30 seconds
Power Walk or Run	30 minutes, Treadmill walk incline of 6-10 for 2 minutes every 3 minutes	30-45 minutes Treadmill jog incline 3-5 for 30 seconds every 5 minutes	30-45 minutes Treadmill jog incline 3-5 for 30 seconds every 5 minutes

DAY 5

Exercises	Beginner	Intermediate	Fit Girl
Jump Rope or Jumping Jacks	1 minute	3 minutes	3 minutes with intermediate high knee running, every 30 seconds for 30 seconds
Squats : Legs	Air squats 50 reps	Air squats 25 reps	Air squats 25 reps
Bicep Curls	Band 30 seconds or 5-10 lb. dumbbells 15 reps	Band 1 minute or 10-20 lb. dumbbells 15 reps	Band 1 minute or 10-20 lb. dumbbells 15 reps
Squats : Legs	Air squats 25 reps	Dumbbell or Bar squats 15 reps w single dumbbell : 15-25 lbs. or 25lb. bar with weight	Dumbbell squats 15 reps w single dumbbell : 15-25 lbs. or 25lb. bar with weight
Bicep Curls	Band 30 seconds or 5-10 lb. dumbbells 15 reps	Band 1 minute or 10-20 lb. dumbbells 15 reps. Best if you **pyramid (drop set) weight, change weight every 5 reps from heaviest to lighter but should challenge you.** Example, 5-8 reps 15lbs drop and do 6-8 more reps with 12lbs. Challenge	Band 1 minute or 10-20 lb. dumbbells 15 reps. Best if you **pyramid (drop set) weight, change weight every 5 reps from heaviest to lighter but should challenge you.** Example, 5-8 reps 15lbs drop and do 6-8 more reps with 12lbs. Challenge yourself

		yourself safely with good form with heavier.	safely with good form with heavier.
Squats : Legs	Air squats 25 reps	Dumbbell or Bar squats 25 reps w single dumbbell : 15-25 lbs. or 25lb. bar with weight. **Pyramid (drop set) weight heavy to light every 5-10 reps**	Dumbbell or Bar squats 25 reps w single dumbbell : 15-25 lbs. or 25lb. bar with weight. **Pyramid (drop set) weight heavy to light every 5-10 reps**
Walking Lunges 20 feet	Rest 1-2 minutes and proceed to plank	2 minute: Holding a dumbbell in each hand, 10-15lbs. Start out with Heaviest weight you can and every 20 feet drop to little lighter	2 minute: Holding a dumbbell in each hand, 10-15lbs. Start out with Heaviest weight you can and every 20 feet drop to little lighter
Bicep Curls	Band 30 seconds or 5-10 lb. dumbbells 15 reps	Band 1 minute or 10-12 lb. dumbbells 15 reps	Band 1 minute or 10-20 lb. dumbbells 15 reps
Squats : Legs Followed by lunge pulses	Air squats 25 reps followed by 10 pulse lunges each leg	Dumbbell or Bar squats 25 reps w single dumbbell : 15-25 lbs. or 25lb. bar with weight. **Pyramid (drop set) weight heavy to light every 5-10 reps followed by 20 pulse lunges each leg**	Dumbbell or Bar squats 25 reps w single dumbbell : 15-25 lbs. or 25lb. bar with weight. **Pyramid (drop set) weight heavy to light every 5-10 reps followed by 25 pulse lunges each leg**

Star Jumps	10 reps	25 reps	25 reps
Bicep Curls	Band 30 seconds or 5-10 lb. dumbbells 15 reps	Band 1 minute or 10-12 lb. dumbbells 15 reps	Band 1 minute or 10-20 lb. dumbbells 15 reps
High Knee Step Ups	10 reps each leg	10 reps each leg holding a dumbbell in each hand 10-20 lb.	10 reps each leg holding a dumbbell in each hand 10-20 lb.
Squat and press (shoulder)	10 reps with 5-10 lbs.	10 reps with 10-15lbs.	10 reps with 10-20 lbs.
High Knee Step Ups	10 reps each leg	10 reps each leg holding a dumbbell in each hand 10-20 lb.	10 reps each leg holding a dumbbell in each hand 10-20 lb.
Back Leg Curl with Fitness Ball	20 reps	30 reps	30 reps
Stand Ups	10 each leg	25 each leg	25 each leg
Bridges	50 reps	100 reps with weight	100 reps with weight
Single Leg Bridges	20 each leg	50 each leg	50 each leg
Jumping squats	20 reps	20 reps holding a dumbbell or medicine ball (15-25lb.) landing and going into full squat and jumping up high with straight legs. Follow with 10 no weight	15-25 reps holding a dumbbell or medicine ball (15-25lb.) landing and going into full squat and jumping up high with straight legs. Follow with 10 no weight

45

Back Leg Curl with Fitness Ball	10 reps	25 reps	25 reps
Bridges	25 reps	100 reps	100 reps
Mile Run	Walk ½ mile and trot ½ mile	Jog ½ mile and 70% sprint ½ mile	Jog ½ mile and 70 % sprint ½ mile
Walk or run	Walk 15-30 minutes. Hill path. If you have a Treadmill walk incline 6-10.	Sprints (rest 30 sec between sets) 3 x 25 yards, 80% max 2 x 50 yards, same 1 x 100 yards, same	Sprints (rest 30 sec between sets) 3 x 25 yards, 80% max 2 x 50 yards, same 1 x 100 yards, same 2 x 50 yards, same

DAY 6

Exercises	Beginner	Intermediate	Fit Girl
Cardio	Power Walk, Bike and/or Run 2-4 miles	Run 4-6 miles Hills included	Run 5-7 miles Hills included
Abs: Knee Tucks	10 reps	25 reps	50 reps
Abs: Plank with walking	Plank with walking, 10 each side	Plank with walking, 30 each side	Plank with walking, 30 each side
Abs: High Plank to Low Plank	10 each side	20 each side	30 each side
Abs: Leg Lifts Leg flutters	20 reps 30 sec	40 reps 1 minute	50 reps 1 minute
Abs: Knee Tucks	15 reps	40 reps	50 reps
Cardio	Jump Rope or Jumping Jacks 2 minutes	Jump Rope or Jumping Jacks 3 minutes	Jump Rope or Jumping Jacks 3 minutes, every 30 seconds high knee running for 30 seconds

DAY 7

Rest and Stretch 20 minutes. Yoga is best.

WEEK 3

Day 1

Exercises	Beginner	Intermediate	Fit Girl
Jump Rope or Jumping Jacks	2 minutes	3 minutes	3 minutes with intermediate high knee running, every 30 seconds for 30 seconds
Squats : Legs	Air squats 50 reps	Air squats 50 reps	Air squats 50 reps
Sissy Squats	50 reps	75 reps	100 reps
Bicycle : Abs	1 minute	2 minutes	2 minutes
Squats	Air squats 40 reps	Dumbbell or Bar squats 15 reps w single dumbbell : 15-30 lbs. or 25lb. bar with weight	Dumbbell squats 15 reps w single dumbbell : 15-30 lbs. or 25lb. bar with weight
Leg Lift flutters: Abs	30 seconds	1 minute	1 minute
Reverse Lunge with kick	10 each leg	20 each leg	25 each leg
Star Jumps	25 reps	50 reps	50 reps
Cardio	Jog ½ mile	Jog 1 mile	Jog 1 mile(1/2 mile sprint)
Squats Followed by pulse lunges	Air squats 40 reps	Dumbbell or Bar squats 15 reps w single dumbbell : 15-25 lbs. or 25lb. bar with weight	Dumbbell squats 15 reps w single dumbbell : 15-35 lbs. or 25lb. bar with weight immediately

		immediately follow each set with 10 pulse lunges each leg	follow each set with 10 pulse lunges each leg
Bicycle : Abs	1 minute	1 minute	1 minute
Cross overs	20 each side	30 each side	30 each side
Reverse Lunge with power jump	10 each leg	20 each leg	25 each leg
Leg lifts, 90 to 3"	25 reps	50 reps	50 reps
Leg Lifts (3" off ground) 1. flutters 2. Criss cross	1. 30 seconds 2. 30 seconds	1. 1 minute 2. 30 seconds	1. 1 minute 2. 30 seconds
Squats	skip	Dumbbell squats 15 reps w single dumbbell : 15-25 lbs. or 25lb. bar with weight immediately follow each set with 10 pulse lunges each leg	Dumbbell squats 15 reps w/ single dumbbell: 15-40 lbs. or 25lb. bar with weight immediately follow each set with 10 pulse lunges each leg
Skating	30 seconds	1 minute	1 minute
Star Jumps	10 reps	40 reps	50 reps
Sissy Squats	25 Reps	50 Reps	50 Reps
Skating	1 minute	2 minutes	2 minutes
Walking Lunges 20 feet	1 minute: Holding no weight	1 minute: Holding 10-15 lb. dumbbells	2 minutes: Holding 10-15 lb. dumbbells
Knee Tucks	10 Reps	25 Reps	25 Reps
Walking	Rest 1-2	1 minute: Holding a	1 minute: Holding a

Exercise Pictorials and Descriptions

Lunges 20 feet	minutes and proceed to plank	dumbbell in each hand, 10-15lbs.	dumbbell in each hand, 10-15lbs.
Skating	Rest	1 minute	1 minute
Knee tucks	10-20 reps	25-50 reps	40-50 reps
Push Ups	10-20 reps	25-50 reps, start no knees	25-50 reps, start no knees
High Plank Arm Pulses	20 reps	50 reps	50-100 reps
Power Walk or Run	15 minutes	15 – 30 minutes	15 – 30 minutes, pick up the pace every other minute for 15 seconds

DAY 2

Exercises	Beginner	Intermediate	Fit Girl
Jump Rope or Jumping Jacks	2 minutes	3 minutes	3 minutes with intermediate high knee running, every 30 seconds for 30 seconds
Bridges	50 reps	50 with weight	50 with weight
One Leg Bridge	20 both side	50 both sides, no weight	50 both side w/ weight
Skating	1 minute	2 minutes	2 minutes
Bridges	50 reps	50 with weight	50 with weight
One Leg Bridge	10 both side	50 both side w/ weight	50 both side w/ weight
Push Ups	10-20 reps	25-40 reps	25-50 reps
Heavy Plie Squats, single dumbbell	15 reps w/ 15 lbs	20 reps w/20-30 lbs.	25 reps w/20-40 lbs.
Plie Pulses (hands on thighs), mid to low level	25 reps	50 reps	50 reps
Bridges	25 reps	50 with weight	50 with weight
Stiff Leg Dead Lifts	10 with light weight 10-12lbs	15 with 10-20 lbs.	20 with 10-20 lbs.
Heavy Plie Squats, single dumbbell	15 reps w/ 15 lbs	20 reps w/20-30 lbs.	25 reps w/20-40 lbs.
Running High Knees	2 minutes	2 minutes	2 minutes
Bridges	25	50 with weight	50 with weight

One Leg Bridge	10 both side	25 both side w/ weight	25 both side w/ weight
Back Leg Curl with Fitness Ball	10 reps	25 reps	25 reps
Swimming	1 minute	2 minutes	2 minutes
Step ups on bench	20 reps each leg	20 reps each leg holding dumbbell in each hand	20 reps each leg holding dumbbell in each hand
Stand Ups	20 each leg	30 each leg	30 each leg
Skating	skip	1 minute	1 minute
Back Leg Curl with Fitness Ball	10 reps	25 reps	25 reps
Stiff Leg Deadlifts with dumbbells	10 reps w/ 5-10 lbs.	10 reps w/15 lbs.	10 reps w/15 lbs.
Swimming	30 seconds	1 minute	2 minutes
Jumping Squat holding a medicine ball or dumbbell	10 reps, 5-10 lb.	15 reps,15-20 lb.	25 reps, 15-30 lb.
Step ups on bench	20 each leg	20 each leg holding dumbbell in each hand	20 each leg holding dumbbell in each hand
Swimming	30 seconds	1 minute	2 minutes
Stand ups	20 each leg	30 each leg	30 each leg
Push Ups w/ or w/out knees	30 seconds	1 minute or till failure	1 minute or till failure
Power Walk or Run	20-30 minutes	20- 30 minutes, pick up the pace every other minute for 15 seconds	20- 30 minutes, pick up the pace every other minute for 15 seconds

DAY 3

Exercises	Beginner	Intermediate	Fit Girl
Jump Rope or Jumping Jacks	2 minute	3 minutes	3 minutes with intermediate high knee running, every 30 seconds for 30 seconds
High Knee Running	2 minute	3 minutes	3 minutes, every 30 seconds perform 20 punches from your face in a boxing position
Alternate Front Kicks, ball of foot	1 minute	2 minutes	2 minutes
Reverse Lunge with kicks	15 reps each side	25 reps each side	30 reps each side
Star Jumps	25 reps	50 reps	50 reps
Mountain Climbers, hit the ground with both balls of feet at same time!	1 minute	2 minutes	2 minutes, every 15 seconds perform 2 push ups
Leg Lifts 3 inches off the ground : Abs	Flutter 15 sec Criss cross 15 sec Repeat both 2x	Flutter 30 sec Criss Cross 30 sec Repeat both 2x	Flutter 30 sec Criss Cross 30 sec Repeat both 2x
45 Degree	10 reps	10 reps, draw in	10 reps, draw in

Crunches		knees and repeat 3x	knees and repeat 4x
Skating	30 seconds	2 minutes	2 minutes
Alternate Front Kicks, ball of foot	1 minute	2 minutes	2 minutes
Leg Lifts: 90 degrees to 3 inches off the ground plus 1. Flutter 2. Criss cross	Leg Lifts: 25 reps 1. Flutter 30 sec 2. Criss cross 30 sec	Leg Lifts 50 reps 1. Flutter 30 sec 2. Criss Cross 30 sec	Leg Lifts 50 reps 1. Flutter 30 sec 2. Criss Cross 30 sec
Push Ups	10 reps	25-50 reps	25-50 reps
Leg Lifts : 90 to 3" Abs	20 reps	50 reps	50 reps
Star Jumps	10 reps	25 reps	50 reps
Jump Rope or Jumping Jacks	1 minute	2 minutes	2 minutes with intermediate high knee running, every 30 seconds for 30 seconds
Skating	30 seconds	1 minute	1 minute holding a dumbbell or medicine ball at chest
Standing Bicep Curls	20 reps, 10-15lbs.	10 reps, 10-12lbs 10 reps 15-20 lbs	10 reps, 10-12lbs 10 reps 15-20 lbs
Hammer curls	15 reps, 5-12 lbs	20 reps, 10-15 lbs.	20 reps, pyramid weight starting with heavy 15-20 lbs

			doing as many as possible and switch to lighter ie. 12lbs.
Walking lunge 20 feet	Holding 5-10 lbs. in each hand	Holding 10-20 lbs. in each hand	Holding 15-25lbs. in each hand
Leg Lifts :90 to 3" Abs	20 reps	50 reps	50 reps
Plank	1 minute with walking feet	1 minute with walking feet	1-2 minutes with walking feet
Standing Bicep curls, curl together	15 reps, 8-12 lbs.	20 reps, pyramid weight starting with heavy 15-20 lbs doing as many as possible and switch to lighter ie. 12lbs.	20 reps, pyramid weight starting with heavy 15-20 lbs doing as many as possible and switch to lighter ie. 12lbs.
High Knee Running	------	1 minute	1 minute, intensity last 30 seconds
Push Ups	------	25-50 reps, start no knees	25-50 reps, start no knees
Standing Bicep Curls with light weight or band	------	30 reps-40 reps with a band or light weight	30-50 reps with a band or light weight
Power Walk or Run	15 minutes	15 – 30 minutes	15 – 30 minutes, pick up the pace every other minute for 15 seconds

DAY 4

Exercises	Beginner	Intermediate	Fit Girl
Jump Rope or Jumping Jacks	1 minute	3 minutes	3 minutes with intermediate high knee running, every 30 seconds for 30 seconds
Star Jumps	10 reps	20 reps	20 reps
Push Ups	10 reps	20 reps	30 reps
Star Jumps	10 reps	50 reps	50 reps
Push Up Pulses	20 reps	50 reps	50 - 100 reps
Burpees	5 reps	40 reps	50 reps
Bicycle : Abs	30 sec - 1 minute	1 minute	2 minutes
Sit ups with a twist	25 reps	25 – 50 reps	25 -50 reps
High Knee Running	1 minute	2 minutes	2 minutes, increase pace for 15 seconds every 30 seconds
9. Push Backs, dumbbells (pyramid) 20 reps light >>15 reps heavier>>10 reps heavier	5lbs>>8lbs>>10lbs	10lbs>>12lbs>>15-20lbs	10lbs>>12lbs>>15-20lbs
10. Push Ups	10 reps	10 reps	10 reps
11. Tricep Bench	10 reps	20 reps	20-30 reps

12. Star Jumps	10 reps	25 reps	25 reps
13. Low to high Plank	10 reps each arm	15 reps each arm	20 reps each arm
Repeat 1 to 4 above as directed before proceeding to bicycle	2 x	3 x	4-5 x
Bicycle : Abs	1 minute	1 minute	1 minute
Knee Tucks : Abs	10 reps	50 reps	50 reps
Jump Rope or Jumping Jacks	1 minute	3 minutes	3 minutes with intermediate high knee running, every 30 seconds for 30 seconds
Power Walk or Run	30 minutes, Treadmill walk incline of 6-10 for 2 minutes every 3 minutes	30-45 minutes Treadmill jog incline 3-5 for 30 seconds every 5 minutes	30-45 minutes Treadmill jog incline 3-5 for 30 seconds every 5 minutes

DAY 5

Exercises	Beginner	Intermediate	Fit Girl
Jump Rope or Jumping Jacks	1 minute	3 minutes	3 minutes with intermediate high knee running, every 30 seconds for 30 seconds
Squats : Legs	Air squats 50 reps	Air squats 25 reps	Air squats 25 reps
Bicep Curls	Band or 5-10 lb. dumbbells, 15 reps	Band or 10-12 lb. dumbbells, 15 reps	Band or 10-12 lb. dumbbells, 15 reps
Squats : Legs	Air squats 50 reps	Dumbbell or Bar squats 20 reps w single dumbbell : 15-25 lbs. or 25lb. bar with weight	Dumbbell squats 20 reps w single dumbbell : 15-25 lbs. or 25lb. bar with weight
Bicep Curls	Band or 5-10 lb. dumbbells 15 reps	Band or 10-12 lb. dumbbells 15 reps. Best if you **pyramid (drop set) weight, change weight every 5 reps from heaviest to lighter but should challenge you.** Example, 5-8 reps 15lbs drop and do 6-8 more reps with 12lbs. Challenge yourself safely with good form with heavier.	Band or 10-12 lb. dumbbells 15 reps. Best if you **pyramid (drop set) weight, change weight every 5 reps from heaviest to lighter but should challenge you.** Example, 5-8 reps 15lbs drop and do 6-8 more reps with 12lbs. Challenge yourself safely with good form with heavier.

Squats : Legs	Dumbbell or Bar Squats 15 reps w single dumbbell: 10-20 lbs.	Dumbbell or Bar squats 25 reps w single dumbbell : 15-25 lbs. or 25lb. bar with weight. **Pyramid (drop set) weight heavy to light every 5-10 reps**	Dumbbell or Bar squats 25 reps w single dumbbell : 15-25 lbs. or 25lb. bar with weight. **Pyramid (drop set) weight heavy to light every 5-10 reps**
Walking Lunges 20 feet	Rest 1-2 minutes and proceed to plank	2 minute: Holding a dumbbell in each hand, 10-15lbs. Start out with Heaviest weight you can and every 20 feet drop to little lighter	2 minute: Holding a dumbbell in each hand, 10-15lbs. Start out with Heaviest weight you can and every 20 feet drop to little lighter
Bicep Curls	Band or 5-10 lb. dumbbells 15 reps	Band or 10-12 lb. dumbbells 15 reps	Band or 10-12 lb. dumbbells 15 reps
Squats : Legs	Dumbbell or Bar Squats 15 reps w single dumbbell: 10-20 lbs.	Dumbbell or Bar squats 25 reps w single dumbbell : 15-25 lbs. or 25lb. bar with weight. **Pyramid (drop set) weight heavy to light every 5-10 reps**	Dumbbell or Bar squats 25 reps w single dumbbell : 15-25 lbs. or 25lb. bar with weight. **Pyramid (drop set) weight heavy to light every 5-10 reps**
Star Jumps	10 reps	25 reps	25 reps
Bicep Curls	Band or 5-10 lb. dumbbells 15 reps	Band or 10-12 lb. dumbbells 15 reps	Band or 10-12 lb. dumbbells 15 reps

Exercise			
Step ups on bench	10 reps each leg	10 reps each leg holding a dumbbell in each hand 10-20 lb.	10 reps each leg holding a dumbbell in each hand 10-20 lb.
Squat and press (shoulder)	15 reps 5-10 lbs. Press dumbbells up when you're moving up. Weights facing your ears.	10 reps with 10-15 lbs. Press dumbbells up when you're moving up. Weights facing your ears.	10 reps with 10-15 lbs. Press dumbbells up when you're moving up. Weights facing your ears.
Step ups on bench	10 reps each leg	10 reps each leg holding a dumbbell in each hand 10-20 lb.	10 reps each leg holding a dumbbell in each hand 10-20 lb.
Back Leg Curl with Fitness Ball	20 reps	30 reps	30 reps
Step ups on bench	10 reps each leg	20 reps each leg holding a dumbbell in each hand 10-20 lb.	30 reps each leg holding a dumbbell in each hand 10-20 lb.
Bridges	50 reps	100 reps with weight	100 reps with weight
Single Leg Bridges	20 each leg	50 each leg	50 each leg
Jumping squats	20 reps	20 reps holding a dumbbell or medicine ball (15-25lb.) landing and going into full squat and jumping up high with	15-25 reps holding a dumbbell or medicine ball (15-25lb.) landing and going into full squat and jumping up high with

		straight legs. Follow with 10 no weight	straight legs. Follow with 10 no weight
Back Leg Curl with Fitness Ball	10 reps	25 reps	25 reps
Bridges	50 reps	100 reps	100 reps
Mile Run	Walk ½ mile and trot ½ mile	Jog ½ mile and 70% sprint ½ mile	Jog ½ mile and 70 % sprint ½ mile
Walk or run	Walk 15-30 minutes. Hill path. If you have a Treadmill walk incline 6-10.	Sprints (rest 30 sec between sets) 3 x 25 yards, 80% max 2 x 50 yards, same 1 x 100 yards, same	Sprints (rest 30 sec between sets) 3 x 25 yards, 80% max 2 x 50 yards, same 1 x 100 yards, same 2 x 50 yards, same

DAY 6

Exercises	Beginner	Intermediate	Fit Girl
Cardio	Power Walk, Bike and/or Run 3-4 miles	Run 4-6 miles Hills included	Run 5-7 miles Hills included
Abs: Knee Tucks	10-15 reps	25-50 reps	50 reps
Abs: Plank with walking	Plank with walking, 15 each side	Plank with walking, 30 each side	Plank with walking, 30 each side
Abs: High Plank to Low Plank	10 each side	20 each side	30 each side
Abs: Leg Lifts (ground to 90 degrees)	25 reps	40 reps	50 reps
Abs: Knee Tucks	15 reps	40 reps	50 reps
Cardio	Sprints 70% max Jog 25 yards> sprint back 70% max> rest 30 seconds and repeat 5x	Sprints 70% max Jog 50 yards> sprint back 70% max> no rest and repeat 6x	Sprints 90-100% max 50 yards> sprint back 90-100%> no rest and repeat 6x (300 yards total)> rest 1 minute after performing 50 yards x 6 and repeat all again.

DAY 7

Exercises	Beginner	Intermediate	Fit Girl
Cardio	Power Walk, Bike and/or Run 3-4 miles	Run 4-6 miles Hills included	Run 5-8 miles Hills included

EXERCISE PICTORIALS AND DESCRIPTIONS:

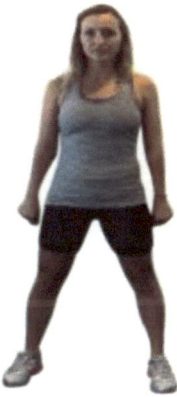

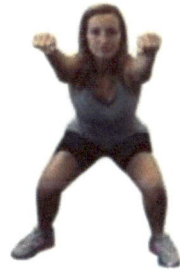

Squat (air squats): best when performed with high reps (25-100), feet hip distance, stand erect, squat down, hips back and hands rise up with arms straight, all weight on back heel, head up or forward with chest up. Press off ground with heel and glutes. Stand and press hips forward while squeezing glutes on top. Repeat. Don't bounce on bottom. You can do small pulses (bottom to midpoint) at the end of all your full reps for an extra burn.

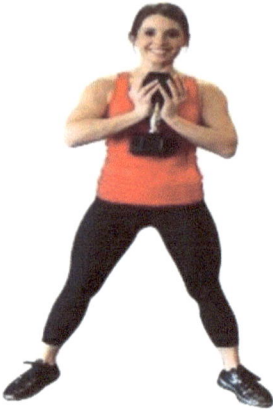

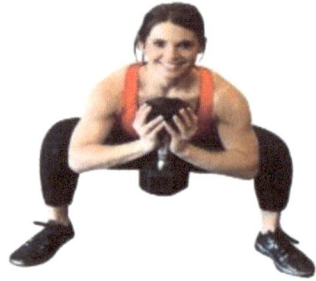

Squat with Dumbbell: Stand erect, feet slightly wider then shoulder, toes out, dumbbell vertical, squat until bum is below parallel unless you have a weak knee or lower back. Stand back up and squeeze glutes and repeat.

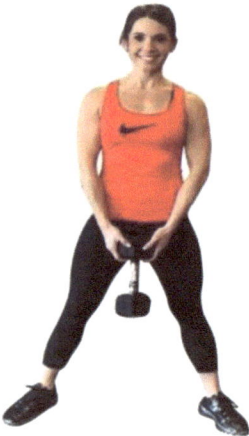

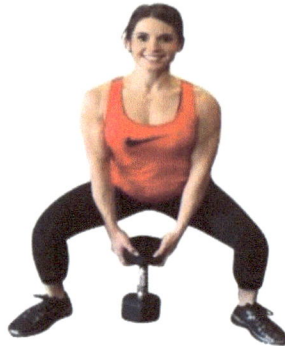

Plie Squat: Stand erect, feet wider then shoulders, feet in plie position, arms locked with dumbbell hanging. Squat down and up. To make extra effective: stop on the bottom and only go half way up and repeat pulsing until failure.

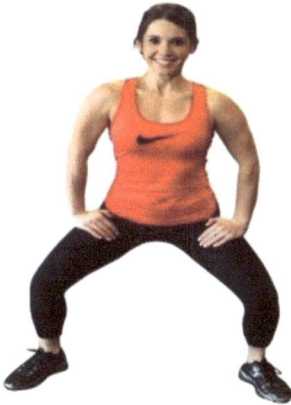

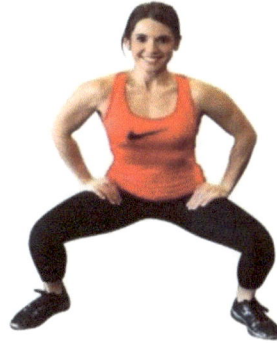

Plie' Pulses: Stand erect, feet wider then shoulder width, feet turned out wide in plie position, palms on upper thigh with fingers pointing down, Squat 2 inches (starting point). Squat down below parallel while pressing hands down hard on thighs (pressure) and rise to starting point (don't stand erect). Continue to pulse start position to below parallel for designated time and/or till failure.

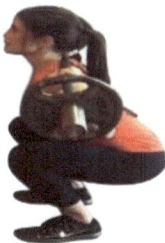

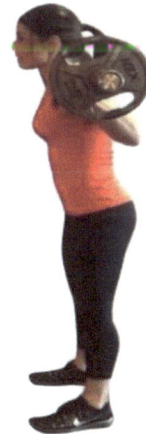

Squat with Bar Bell: Stand erect, bar across upper shoulder blade not on neck, feet hip distance apart, toes turned slightly out, weight on heels, sit and squat with chest up and looking slightly forward, bum goes parallel or slightly below parallel from floor. Drive off heels while looking up and stand. Pause and repeat for reps. Best with spotter and never with prior injury.

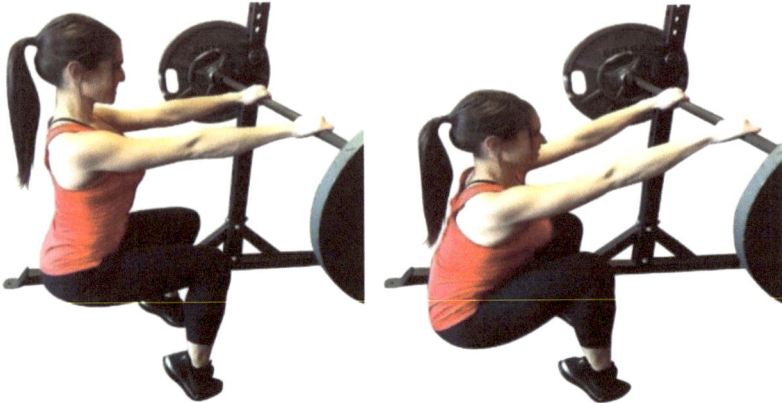

Sissy Squats: Holding onto a very secure bar or handle, place feet hip distance apart or heels together and toes out, rise heels off the ground so you are on the balls of your feet the entire time, hold with hands at eye level, lock out arms and lean back with feet almost under your hands, all pressure should be on front legs in squat position, hold with arms straight and squat from midway point down until your bum is 3-5 inches under your knee point. Rise up to midpoint and repeat for desired time or reps.

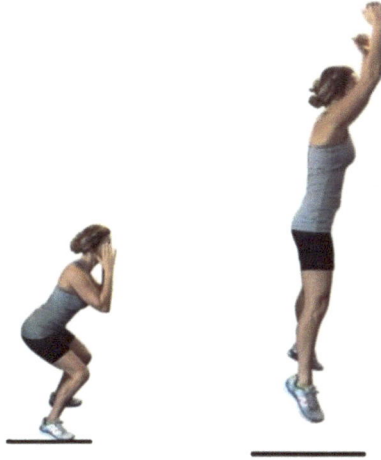

Jumping Squat: Squat position, bum back and back 45 degrees, pressure on heels, elbows in, hands facing ears, press off the ground hard with toes while locking arms high overhead, make sure knees lock out and land soft onto ground. Pause and squat to repeat. Don't jump up without good form.

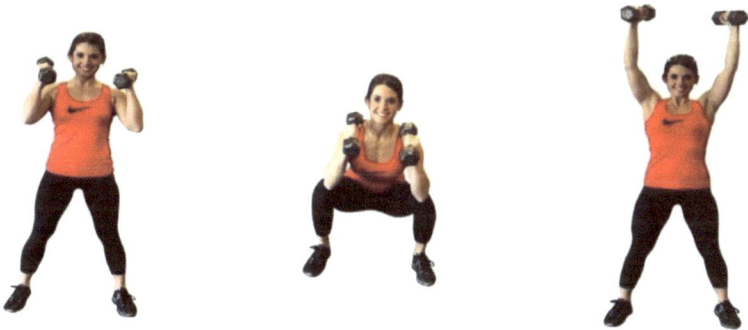

Squat and Press: Start erect with dumbbells vertical over shoulders. Squat with weight back on heels. Stand up and press at the same time over head. Bring weight back down slowly to shoulder and repeat.

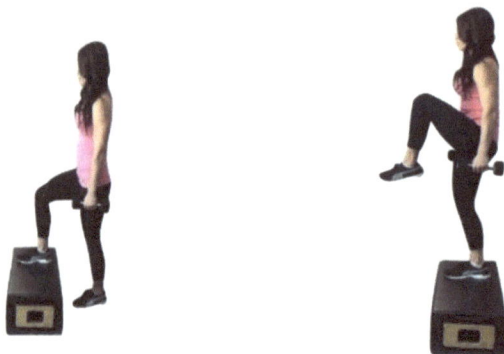

High Knee Step Ups: Place foot on bench or high step. Make sure when foot is on bench the knee is not higher than your hip. Hold dumbbells or place hands behind head. Push Off heel on bench to stand up tall so bent legs knee locks out when you stand up. Raise knee high or just stand on bench next to other leg. Step down with foot that came up. Keep foot on bench entire time until the reps are completely finished. To make more challenging you can kick your foot out once you bring the knee high (front kick).

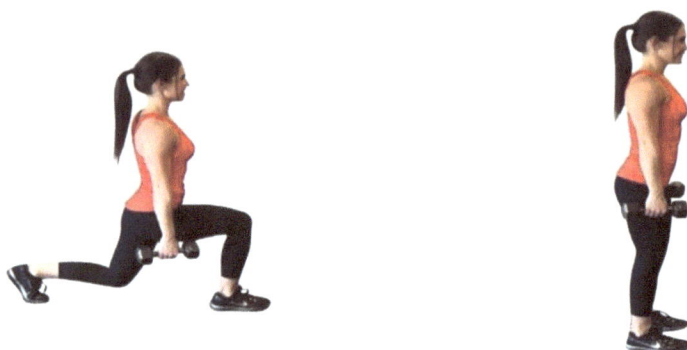

Stationary Lunge: stand erect holding dumbbells (make sure dumbbells are tilting back never forward) in each hand or place hands on hips or behind head. Feet hip distance apart as normal walking. Step out onto front heel not toe. Make sure back knee goes down 90 degrees and front knee stays behind front toe. Back knee should drop straight down until inch off ground. Push off front heel back to stand erect and repeat for the same leg as directed for reps on plan. Switch feet and repeat.

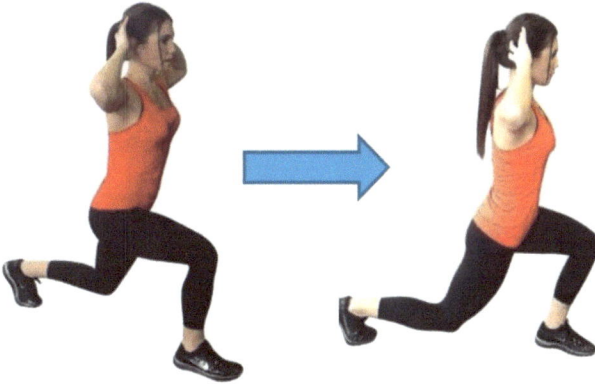

Walking lunge: Same technique as above but you'll walk from right lunge to left lunge in forward position. Bring feet to parallel before stepping forward.

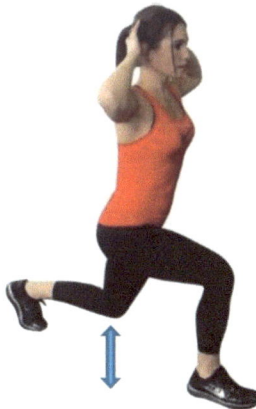

Lunge Pulses: Start in lunge position (see below). Pulse up and down (back knee 1 inch from ground to 3 inches off ground and back to 1 inch, repeat pulsing manner). Stay in same stance for reps on plan. Then switch legs. Hold weight or place hands behind head or on hips.

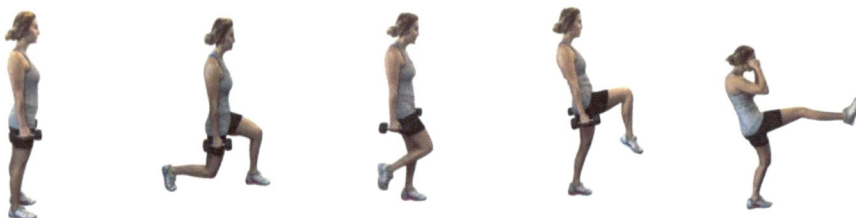

Reverse Lunge with Kick: Standing straight, step back to a reverse lunge, holding weight or hands up on face in a fighting position. Once in lunge position bring leg up to a high knee and lean back while thrusting kick out with pointed foot and ball off foot. Best if you can kick a bag with the ball of foot. Repeat on same side as indicated by your plan. Switch to other leg and repeat the same.

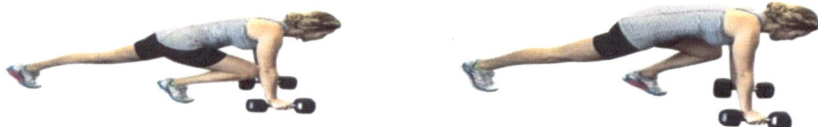

Mountain Climbers: place hands on sturdy dumbbells for less pressure on wrist or on the ground. Make sure you drop hips slightly lower than your shoulders. Keep stomach in tight entire time while simultaneously driving the right foot up to chest while driving the left foot back. Make sure both balls of feet drive into the ground. Don't allow front foot to just stay dangling in the air. You want to drive up and back as if going up a mountain through mud. You should here a thump from both feet hitting. Increase speed with good form. Don't slouch.

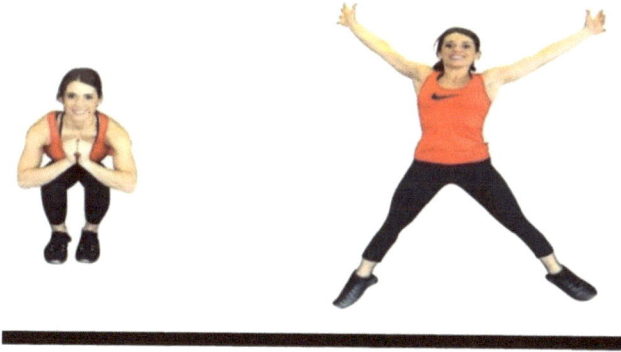

Star Jumps: start in tuck position with hands under chin, feet and knees together as if downhill skiing, spring hard off toes straight up into air while straightening both your legs and arms out wide. Hands and arms go straight up and out not out and up. Land soft onto ground into starting (tuck position). Repeat.

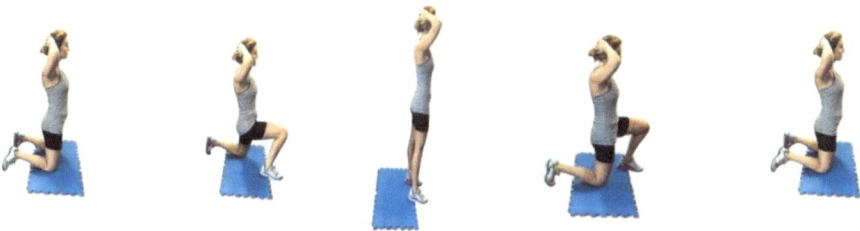

Stand Ups: Right side example. Start with both knees down, Step straight up with right foot, hips forward entire time, don't step out to the side (make sure step directly in front as if lunging), stand up and now go back to start position by dropping right knee first then the left knee. Notice she steps up on right and down with right. She would do this for the reps required before doing the same with left side. Hold hands behind head or hold a weight (dumbbell or medicine ball).

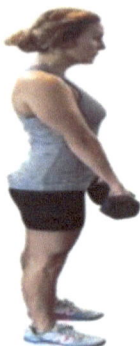

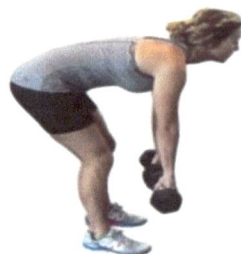

Stiff Leg Dead lifts (good mornings): stand up tall, slight bend in knees, with feet hip distance apart. Heels elevated 2 inches or flat. Weights directly in front, perpendicular to legs. Pull Shoulders back and tuck belly in tight. Look up and keep a flatter back while reaching down and out in order to stetch hamstrings. Reach down towards toes and looking up, squeeze glutes and stand up tall (throw ups forward on top) and squeeze glutes. Repeat.

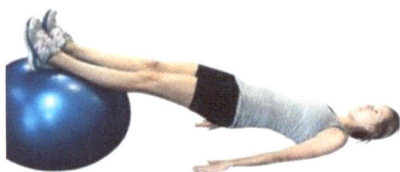

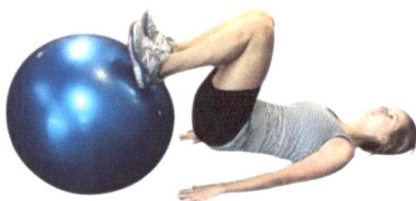

Back Leg Curls with fitness ball: lye in supine position with arms out to side, palms facing down. Place feet up on ball with toes pulled back (flexed) the entire time. Lift hips off the ground the entire exercise. Pull heels towards your bum to roll ball in and then extend legs out. You should feel your hamstrings.

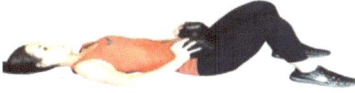

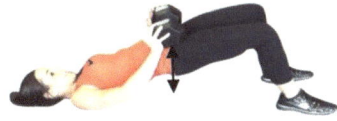

Bridges: lye on back with heels hip distance apart and toes turned out slightly. Place arms by side or a heavy dumbbell on upper thigh and pelvis (keep in place with hands). Press off ground with heels and squeeze glutes to throw hips high into air. Squeeze glutes on top and slowly go back to ground and repeat. You may finish at the end with pulses on top (25-50 extra small reps).

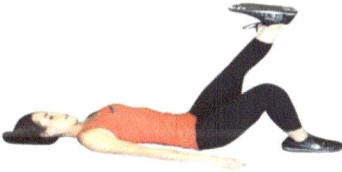

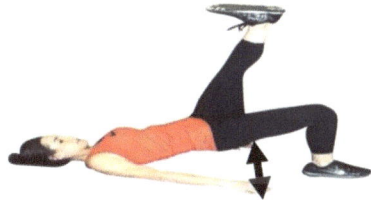

One Leg Bridges: place the heel on the ground directly in alignment with the sit bone. Foot Straight and press off that heel in order for the leg which is straight up and toes flexed goes up as if you're placing your heel on the ceiling. Slowly descend to ground and repeat or keep glutes off the ground an inch the entire time.

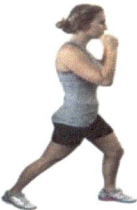

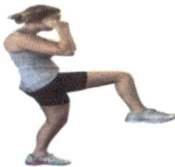

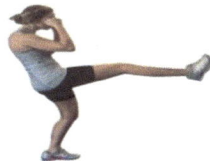

Switch Kicks: get into fighting stance (fist on chin, elbows tight to ribs, feet hip distance apart, front shoulder facing opponent, slight bend in knees and on balls of feet), bring back knee up and snap foot out with ball of foot. Place back to starting position and quickly switch your stance to the back foot is now the front foot and again kick with the back foot on the other side. Switch back and forth with a kick and repeat for reps or time on plan. Best to kick bag with ball of the foot for best cardio burn and leg sculpting. Work on form but perform quickly.

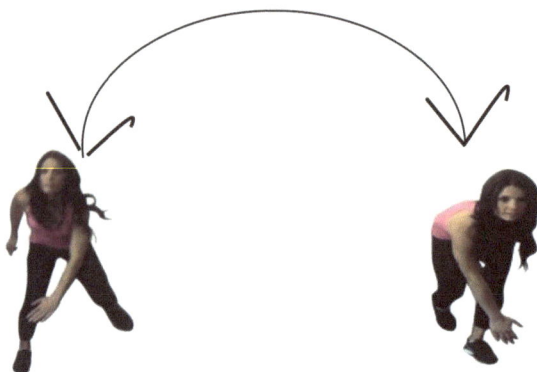

Skating: start in a tuck position. Press off right foot and right leg to spring over to the left. Reach opposite hand to opposite foot while stepping right foot to left foot when you land. Repeat same going the other direction. Key: stay in crouch position entire time in slight forward position so that all pressure is on legs and bum. Go right to left and left to right quickly for time on plan. Push hard and make sure to tap ground with opposite hand.

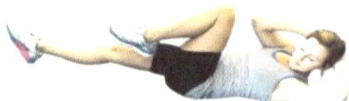

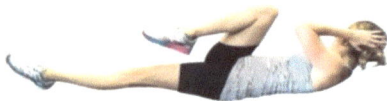

Bicycle: start <u>flexed up</u> in crunch with hands behind ears, elbows wide, knees bent, feet off ground with pointed toe. Draw one knee back while twisting opposite elbow and shoulder towards that knee, simultaneously kick other leg straight out with pointed toes. Make sure to lock out knees and point toes like laser beams going through them. Scrape legs together as they go in and out. Stay in crunch entire time (pressure on abs) and keep elbows and back wide. All the motion happens with a twist. Repeat back and forth for time on plan.

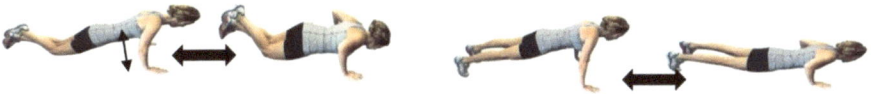

Push Ups (knees or feet): hands slightly wider then shoulder width, fingers facing forward and thumbs in line with under arm. Shoulder slightly forward of hands. Pull in navel while going down and contract triceps, chest and lats (sides of back) to press back up. Lock up on top and repeat.

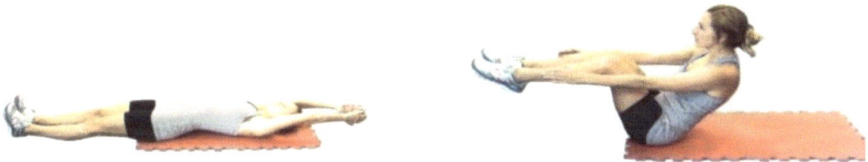

Knee Tucks: Start with arms long over head and hands 2-3 inches from ground. Wide through the shoulders, legs together and abs engaged with breadth by pulling ribs in. Bring arms up and forward while tucking knees to chest and sit up with arms straight out. Slowly go back to starting position. Repeat as on plan.

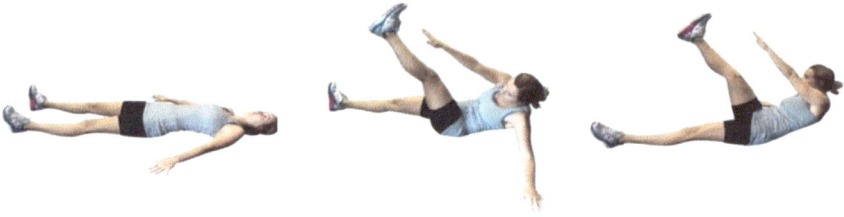

Cross Over: lie flat with feet and hands wider then shoulder width apart. Press off hand to reach other hand to leg that cross overs to opposite foot in the middle while sitting up. **Note:** you can also place one arm out at shoulder height and the opposite arm wide and over the head to reach up and across, the picture above shows both hands and arms by the side. I recommend placing one arm out to side, palm down and the other arm overhead and wide. Repeat all reps on one side before moving onto the other side.

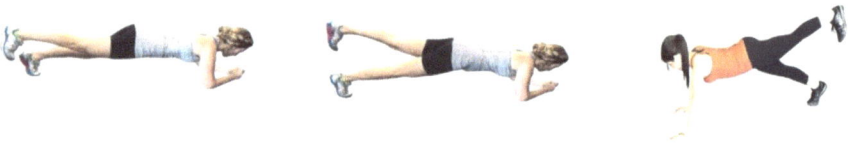

Plank: place forearms directly straight in front of each shoulder or as seen in pic. Best with forearms straight out and palms down. Keep feet hip distance apart pushing back on heels. Shoulders directly in line with hips and ankle (straight line). Keep navel pulled up the entire time.

Plank with walking (low on forearms or high plank on hands): same as plank but you will squeeze your bum before lifting one foot up at a time in a marching manner. Make sure toes are flexed (pulled towards you) the entire time. Squeeze glutes tightly so that your leg (locked out) goes up 3 inches from the ground. Repeat as stated in the plan.

High Plank: same as plank but you will be up on hands with your hands directly under each shoulder.

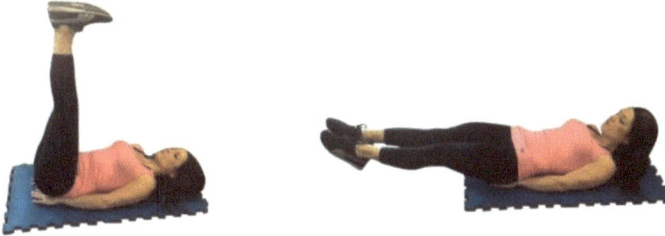

Leg Lifts: start with legs 90 degrees from ground. Lower legs down to 3 inches off the ground (6 inches if you are a beginner or your lower back is week). Hold on bottom 2 inches and bring back to 90 degrees. You may keep your chin tucked looking over feet the entire time with hands under your lower back for support (advanced may stay in a crunch position the entire time with hands behind the head). Repeat as stated. Stop immediately if you feel a strain in lower abs.

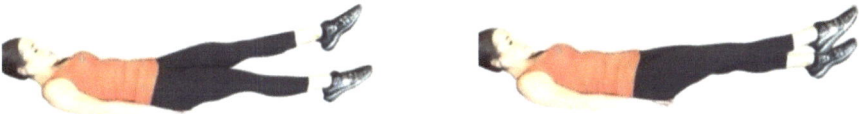

Flutters: start with hands under you lower back and glutes (palms down) for support. Lock knees out entire time and point toes as if laser beams are going through toes. Always, flex legs and lock knees as this will help keep pressure on abs and off lower back. Flutter feet 2-3 inches up and down for time on plan. Head up if you have strong neck muscles and chin down looking over toes entire time.

Criss Cross: with feet 3 inches off the ground, bring one foot over the other in a criss cross manner (one below and 1 above) Scissor lateral. Make sure feet are straight and legs locked as above.

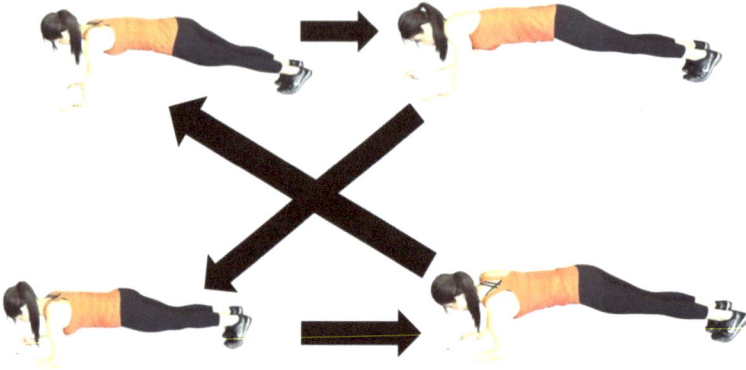

Low to High Plank: (right hand example) start on hands, drop down to right forearm, drop down to left forearm, rise up on right hand, rise up on left hand (back to start). Repeat for reps on plan then do the same for the opposite hand **(left side):** start on hands, drop down to left forearm, drop down to right forearm, rise up on left hand, rise up on right hand (back to start). Repeat for reps on plan.

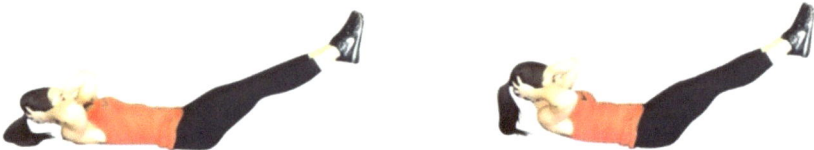

45 Degree Crunches: start with legs up 90 degrees toward ceiling. Place hands behind ears and flex up (crunch) hard to engage abs. Keeping abs engaged now lower legs to 45 degrees (toes pointed and legs locked out straight). Begin to do small crunches always looking over feet the entire time (not up at ceiling). Repeat until your lower back fatigues and repeat for reps or time in plan.

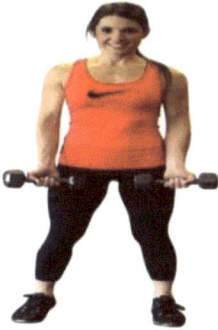

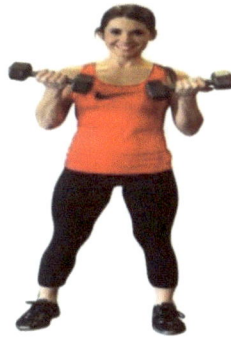

Standing Bicep Curls: stand up tall holding weights with palms up. Back of hand and pinky on thigh so when you curl up it goes directly in front of your shoulder. Squeeze bicep on top and slowly go back to start and repeat.

Standing Band Curls: do same as above but step on middle of band to create tension in band to curl. Recommended band: blue, red or black (blue and black will be most challenging).

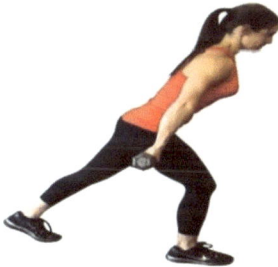

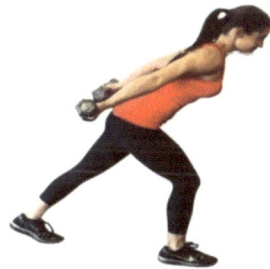

Tricep Push Backs: lean over with one leg forward for support. Arms long, palms up and elbows locked by your side. Start at hip and press back using the back of your arms and upper back muscles. Press to top and hold 2 seconds before lowering (don't lower to middle thigh, keep at hip bone). Make sure to press up and back against gravity. Pulses: hold on top and lower only an inch and press back up in pulsing manner. Always keep palms facing back.

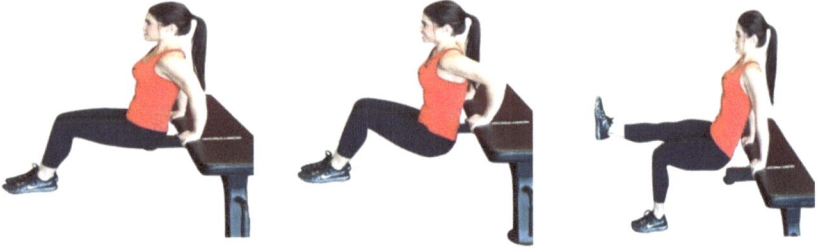

Tricep Bench: using a sturdy chair or bench. Place hands on edge with finger over side. Put feet straight out with feet flat and knees bent not straight (places pressure on shoulder). Go straight down with lower back skimming edge of bench entire the time. Press up by squeezing triceps and lock out elbows on top (contracting triceps). Repeat for reps on plan. **Advanced** you can do equal numbers with the right leg up and then the left leg **or** you can place a heavy dumbbell on your thighs.

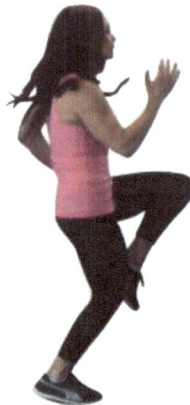

High Knee Running: Run with intensity in place. Feet on fire. Bring up knees high (hip height). Draw knee up as you bring the opposite hand and bent arm up in a pendulum manner. Elbows bent and your arms swing in opposite rhythm. This will help you run with intensity and engage your abs.

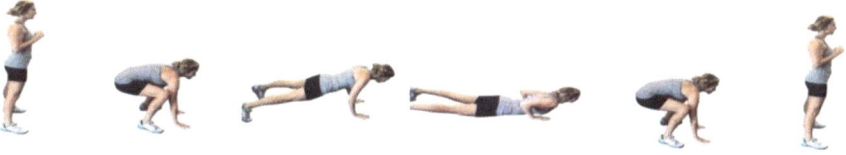

Burpees (down ups): stand erect, squat down and place palms down on ground in front, kick back legs, drop entire body to the ground (rest body), press up hard using upper body while thrown feet under you to land in squat position. Stand up erect and **jump up or perform a star jump**. Repeat.

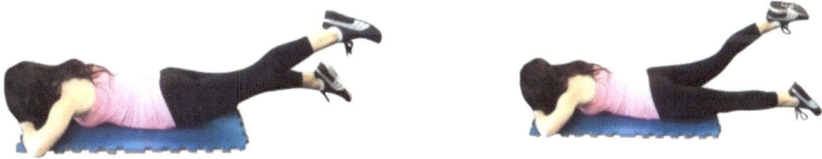

Swimming: lying flat, prone position with your nose placed into triangle created by placing one hand over the other (thumbs and index fingers creating triangle). Pull up nave and straighten legs behind you with toes pointed away. Raise one leg up at a time (lifting thighs).

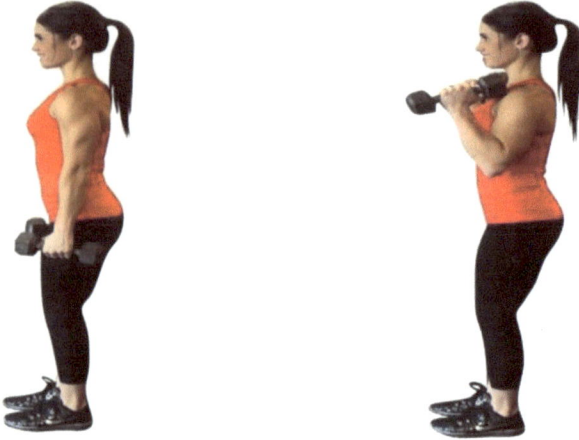

Hammer Curls: Elbows tight to side, feet together, dumbbells vertical. Contract bicep and curl up so that the head of dumbbell goes directly in front of the shoulder. Lower slowly with resistance and repeat.

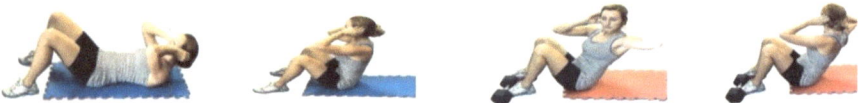

- Sit Up with Twisting: start in a crunch position! (flexed up and looking over knees). Sit up to top in a neutral position. Now twist right and twist left. The keys to performing an effective and safe sit ups:
- Start in a crunch position (engaged abs). When you roll down one vertebrae at a time, land in the same crunch position.
- Don't let head snap back. Keep chin down and look over knees the entire time.
- Go down very slow. Resisting the descend using your abs.

- Twisting make sure your ribs are lifted and elbows out wide. Twist right, go to center then twist left, then go to center and then descend. Lift rib cage when twisting. Don't hunch over.
- Place feet under a heavy dumbbell or secure support to help you keep your feet on the floor while performing the sit up.

SUMMARY:

Hey, Doug Bennett here. I hope you are beginning to love these workouts. My mission since creating my first app, Fitgirl App, has been to help women just like you get amazing workouts without paying thousands to love your results.

If you have any questions or comments. Please don't hesistate to send me an email to bsstudio@comcast.net. Subject: Pocket Trainer for legs.

Check out my other books for more help:

Click on the book link to learn more.

For You:

21 Day Happy Girl Diet and Fitness Plan

21 Day Total Body Tone Up and Diet Guide

Comfort Foods Gone Fit: Recipe Makeovers for your family

For Him:

The Buff Body Blueprint

Fit Actions for Guys To Get and Stay Fit Forever

To Get Free Health Tips, Workouts and Recipes tap on the link below and subscribe today!

Free workouts and Recipes Weekly

---

www.ingramcontent.com/pod-product-compliance
Lightning Source LLC
Chambersburg PA
CBHW040513290326
41930CB00036B/112